The Ultimate Keto Breakfast Cookbook for Women over 50

50 Fast and Delicious Recipes to Burn Fat and Stay Healthy

Katie Attanasio

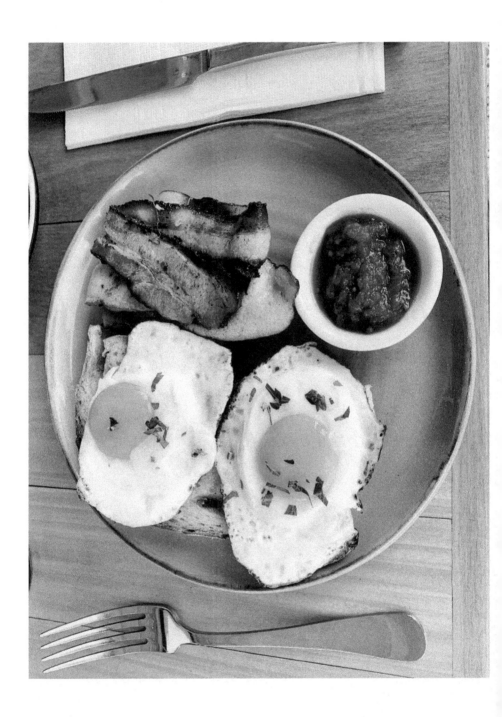

© Copyright 2021 - All rights reserved.

sources. Please consult a licensed professional before attempting any techniques outlined in this book.

By reading this document, the reader agrees that under no circumstances is the author responsible for any losses, direct or indirect, which are incurred as a result of the use of information contained within this document, including, but not limited to, — errors, omissions, or inaccuracies.

Table of Contents

50 Keto Breakfast Recipes

1   Keto Breakfast Brownie Muffins

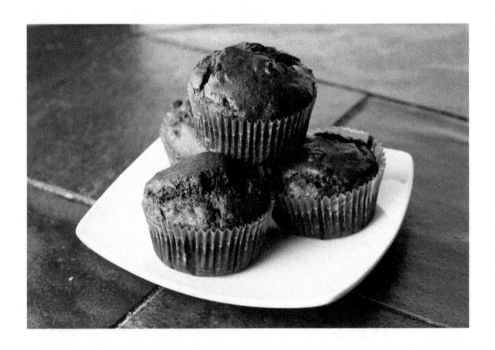

Servings: 6 | **Time:** 20 mins | **Difficulty:** Easy

Nutrients per serving: Calories: 193 kcal | Fat: 14.09g | Carbohydrates: 4.37g | Protein: 6.98g | Fiber: 7.18g

Ingredients

1/4 Cup Caramel Syrup (Sugar-Free)

1 Cup Golden Flaxseed Meal

1/4 Cup Cocoa Powder

1/2 Tbsp. Baking Powder

1/4 Cup Almonds, Slivered

1 Tsp. Vanilla Extract

1/2 Cup Pumpkin Puree

1/2 Tsp. Salt

1 Tsp. Apple Cider Vinegar

1 Egg

1 Tbsp. Cinnamon

2 Tbsps. Coconut Oil

Method

1.   Preheat the oven to 350 degrees F.

2.   Combine all ingredients in a bowl except slivered almonds and whisk well to make a smooth batter.

3.   Put 1/4 cup of the batter in a lined muffin tin and sprinkle the slivered almonds on top.

4.   Put in the preheated oven and bake for about 15 minutes or until cooked through.

2   Keto Breakfast Tacos

Servings: 3 | **Time:** 15 mins | **Difficulty**: Easy

Nutrients per serving: Calories: 443.67 kcal | Fat: 35.68g | Carbohydrates: 2.38g | Protein: 26.41g | Fiber: 1.53g

Ingredients

1/2 Small Avocado

Salt, To Taste

6 Eggs

2 Tbsps. Cheddar Cheese, Shredded

Black Pepper, To Taste

1 Cup Mozzarella Cheese, Shredded

3 Bacon Strips, Cooked

2 Tbsps. Butter

Method

1.   Take a non-stick pan and heat 1/3 cup of mozzarella cheese on it for 2-3 minutes, over medium flame.

2.   Once the cheese becomes golden brown at the edges, lift it with tongs and put on the back of a wooden spoon.

3.   Repeat these steps to make 2 other taco shells like this.

4.   Heat butter in a pan and make scrambled eggs with salt and pepper seasoning, as you like it.

5.   Divide the scrambled eggs, bacon, and avocado into three parts and put on each hardened taco shell.

6.   Sprinkle the shredded cheddar cheese on their top before serving.

3   Breakfast Keto Pizza Waffles

Servings: 2 | **Time**: 15 mins | **Difficulty**: Easy

Nutrients per serving: Calories: 604 kcal | Fat: 48.14g | Carbohydrates: 7.59g | Protein: 30.65g | Fiber: 5.5g

Ingredients

1 Tbsp. Bacon Fat

1/2 Cup Tomato Sauce

4 Eggs

4 Tbsps. Parmesan Cheese, Grated

1 Tsp. Italian Seasoning

3 Tbsps. Almond Flour

1/3 Cup Cheddar Cheese

14 Slices Pepperoni (Optional)

1 Tbsp. Psyllium Husk Powder

1 Tsp. Baking Powder

Salt, To Taste

Black Pepper, To Taste

Method

1. Preheat the waffle iron.

2. Combine all the ingredients (except cheese and tomato sauce) in a bowl and blend using an immersion blender until the mixture thickens.

3. Pour half of the mixture in the waffle iron and close it. Cook until the waffles become golden brown in color. Repeat it for the other half.

4. Top the waffles with tomato sauce and shredded cheese and broil them for 3-5 minutes or until the cheese melts. Add pepperoni to the top if you want.

4   Keto Breakfast Burger

Servings: 2 | **Time**: 30 mins | **Difficulty**: Easy

Nutrients per serving: Calories: 481 kcal | Fat: 37.97g | Carbohydrates: 1.28g | Protein: 31.76g | Fiber: 0.5g

Ingredients

1 Tbsp. Butter, Melted

1 Tbsp. Peanut Butter Powder

Salt, To Taste

4 Bacon Slices, Cooked

1/4 Cup Pepper jack Cheese, Shredded

Black Pepper, To Taste

2 Eggs

1/2 Cup Sausage

Method

1.   Combine the melted butter with peanut butter powder in a bowl and mix well. Set it aside.

2.   Chop the cooked bacon and shape into sausage patties. Fry the patties in a pan until become golden brown on both sides.

3.   Put the cheese on the patties and cover the pan at low heat until the cheese melts.

4.   Take out of the pan and put in a serving plate.

5.   Whisk the egg in a bowl with seasonings and fry it in a non-stick pan.

6.   Put the egg over the patties' cheese and top with peanut butter mixture.

5   Jalapeno Cheddar Waffles

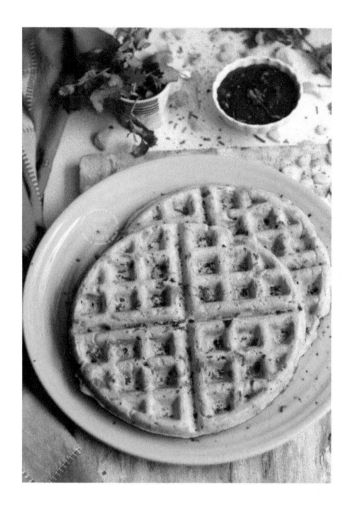

Servings: 2 | **Time:** 10 mins | **Difficulty:** Easy

Nutrients per serving: Calories: 334 kcal | Fat: 27.28g | Carbohydrates: 4.88g | Protein: 15.84g | Fiber: 2.87g

Ingredients

3 Eggs

Salt, To Taste

2 Tbsps. Cheddar Cheese, Shredded

1 Jalapeno

1 Tsp. Baking Powder

1 Tbsp. Coconut Flour

1/3 Cup Cream Cheese

Black Pepper, To Taste

1 Tsp. Psyllium Husk Powder

Method

1. Preheat the waffle iron.

2. Combine all the ingredients in a bowl and blend using an immersion blender until the batter becomes smooth.

3. Pour the batter in the waffle iron and close it.

4. Cook until the waffles become golden brown in color, about 5-6 minutes.

5. Put a low carb topping and serve.

6   Mini Keto Pancake Donuts

Servings: 22 | **Time**: 8 mins | **Difficulty**: Easy

Nutrients per serving: Calories: 32.32 kcal | Fat: 2.68g | Carbohydrates: 0.53g| Protein: 1.41g | Fiber: 0.27g

Ingredients

1/3 Cup Cream Cheese

4 Tbsps. Erythritol

3 Eggs

1 Tsp. Baking Powder

4 Tbsps. Almond Flour

10 Drops Liquid Stevia

1 Tsp. Vanilla Extract

1 Tbsp. Coconut Flour

Method

1.   Preheat a donut maker and spray it with coconut oil spray.

2.   Combine all the ingredients in a bowl and blend using an immersion blender until the mixture becomes smooth.

3.   Pour the batter in each well and cook until become golden brown in color, for about 3 minutes on each side.

4.   Take out and make donuts similarly with the remaining batter.

7   Bacon Cheddar Chive Omelet

Servings: 1 | **Time**: 10 mins | **Difficulty:** Easy

Nutrients per serving: Calories: 386 kcal | Fat: 30.25g | Carbohydrates: 1.86g | Protein: 24.86g | Fiber: 0g

Ingredients

2 Eggs

2 Tbsps. Cheddar Cheese, Shredded

Black Pepper, To Taste

2 Bacon Slices, Cooked

Salt, To Taste

1 Tsp. Chives, Chopped

1 Tsp. Bacon Fat

Method

1.   Crack the eggs in a bowl and season with salt, pepper and chopped chives, whisk well.

2. Take a pan and heat the bacon fat in it over medium-low heat. Pour the egg mixture in it.

3. When the egg sets, add the bacon in its middle. Cook the omelet until done and take the pan off the heat.

4. Sprinkle the shredded cheese on top of the bacon and fold the omelet around it.

8   Keto Peanut Pancakes

Servings: 2 | **Time:** 35 mins | **Difficulty**: Easy

Nutrients per serving: Calories: 744 kcal | Fat: 72.79g | Carbohydrates: 6.61g | Protein: 16.83g | Fiber: 5.15g

Ingredients

1 Egg

1/2 Tsp. Baking Powder

1/4 Tsp. Coconut Oil

1/4 Cup Almond Milk

3 & 1/2 Tbsps. Shelled Peanuts

1/2 Cup Almond Flour

1/2 Tsp. Vanilla Extract

1/4 Cup Heavy Whipping Cream

1/2 Tsp. Stevia

Salt, To Taste

7 Drops Liquid Sucralose

1 Tbsp. Butter, Unsalted & Softened

1/2 Tsp. Baking Soda

Method

1.   Pour heavy cream in a small saucepan and add 2 drops of liquid sucralose, heat them, and stir until combined and thickened. Set this condensed milk aside.

2.   Roast the peanuts in a pan until they become brown. Then grind them with some salt and stevia. Set aside.

3.   Combine the egg, liquid sucralose, almond milk, and vanilla extract in a bowl and whisk well, slowly add the almond flour, baking powder, baking soda, and 1/8 tsp salt in it. Whisk until combined.

4.   Heat some coconut oil in a pan and once it melts pour spoonful of the pancake mixture in it and spread evenly with the back of the spoon. Cook the pancake on both sides until become golden.

5.   Repeat this to make other pancakes.

6.   Transfer the pancakes on plates, spread the condensed milk and softened butter on top of each pancake.

7.   Sprinkle the ground peanuts on top and serve.

9   Bacon Avocado Muffins

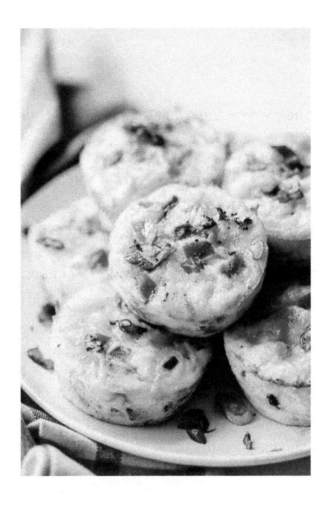

Servings: 16 | **Time:** 55 mins | **Difficulty:** Easy

Nutrients per serving: Calories: 144.19 kcal | Fat: 11.81g | Carbohydrates: 1.71g | Protein: 6.22g | Fiber: 2.66g

Ingredients

2 Tbsps. Butter

2 Avocados, Diced

5 Eggs

3 Spring Onions, Chopped

1 Tsp. Garlic, Minced

5 Bacon Slices

1/2 Cup Almond Flour

1 Tsp. Chives, Dried

1/4 Cup Flaxseed Meal

Salt, To Taste

1 & 1/2 Tbsps. Psyllium Husk Powder

1 Tsp. Cilantro, Dried

2/3 Cup Colby Jack Cheese, Grated

1 Tsp. Baking Powder

1 & 1/2 Tbsps. Lemon Juice

1 & 1/2 Cup Coconut Milk

1/4 Tsp. Red Chili Flakes

Black Pepper, To Taste

Method

1.   Preheat the oven to 350 degrees F.

2.   Combine the eggs, lemon juice, almond flour, coconut milk, flaxseed meal, psyllium husk powder, and spices in a bowl and whisk well to make smooth batter. Cover it and set aside.

3.   Fry the bacon slices in a non-stick pan over medium-low heat, until become crispy.

4.   Add in the butter, spring onions, cheese, and baking powder when the slices are almost done.

5.   Stir fry them while crumbling the bacon with the spoon. Add this mixture to the batter with diced avocados and mix well.

6.   Brush a muffin tin with oil and put the batter in each cup.

7.   Put it in the preheated oven and bake for 24-26 minutes.

10   Raspberry Brie Grilled Waffles

Servings: 2 | **Time**: 15 mins | **Difficulty**: Easy

Nutrients per serving: Calories: 551.5 kcal | Fat: 45.46g | Carbohydrates: 8.71g | Protein: 22.29g | Fiber: 6.8g

Ingredients

The Waffles:

1/2 Cup Almond Flour

2 Tbsps. Flaxseed Meal

1/3 Cup Coconut Milk

1 Tsp. Vanilla Extract

1 Tsp. Baking Powder

2 Eggs

2 Tbsps. Swerve

7 Drops Liquid Stevia

The Filling:

1/2 Cup Raspberries

1 Tsp. Lemon Zest

1 Tbsp. Lemon Juice

2 Tbsps. Butter

1 Tbsp. Swerve

1/3 Cup Brie, Double Cream

Method

1.   Take a pan and brown the butter and swerve in it, then add the raspberries, lemon juice and zest in it. Cook them until everything is heated through. Set this raspberry compote aside.

2.   Preheat the waffle iron.

3.   Combine all the waffle ingredients in a bowl and blend it until a smooth batter is formed.

4.   Pour it on the waffle iron. Cook until both sides become golden brown. Transfer to a dish having brie slices.

5.   Broil them for a few minutes and then serve with raspberry compote on top.

11   Pumpkin Spiced French Toast

Servings: 2 | **Time:** 15 mins | **Difficulty:** Easy

Nutrients per serving: Calories: 429.73 kcal | Fat: 36.7g | Carbohydrates: 7.33g | Protein: 13.36g | Fiber: 9.02g

Ingredients

2 Tbsps. Butter

2 Tbsps. Cream

1/8 Tsp. Orange Extract

1/4 Tsp. Pumpkin Pie Spice

1/2 Tsp. Vanilla Extract

1 Egg

4 Pumpkin Bread Slices

Method

1.   Combine all the ingredients in a bowl except the bread and butter and mix them well.

2.   Put the bread slices in this mixture and let it soak the mixture.

3.   Melt the butter in pan and fry the soaked bread slices in it. Cook both sides until become golden brown.

4.   Transfer to plate and serve with keto toppings.

12   Keto Pumpkin Bread Loaf

Servings: 10 slices | **Time:** 1 hr. 45 mins | **Difficulty**: Easy

Nutrients per serving: Calories: 117.96 kcal | Fat: 8.69g | Carbohydrates: 3.23g | Protein: 4.83g | Fiber: 4.45g

Ingredients

1 & 1/2 Tsps. Pumpkin Pie Spice

3 Egg Whites

1/2 Cup Coconut Milk

1/2 Cup Pumpkin Puree

1 & 1/2 Cup Almond Flour

1/4 Cup Swerve

1/4 Cup Psyllium Husk Powder

1/2 Tsp. Kosher Salt

2 Tsps. Baking Powder

Method

1.   Preheat the oven to 350 degrees F.

2.   Combine all the ingredients in a bowl and whisk/beat well to make a smooth dough, without lumps.

3.   Brush a loaf pan with butter or oil and put the dough in it.

4.   Put in the preheated oven and bake for 1 hour and 15 minutes.

5.   Once done, let cool, slice it and serve.

13   Breakfast Cauliflower Waffles

Servings: 4 | **Time:** 35 mins | **Difficulty**: Easy

Nutrients per serving (half waffle): Calories: 181.5 kcal | Fat: 12.59g | Carbohydrates: 2.86g | Protein: 13.43g | Fiber: 0.98g

Ingredients

2 Tbsp. Butter

1/4 Cup Sour Cream

2 Cups Pork, Pulled

1 Tbsp. Psyllium Husk

2 Tbsps. Golden Flaxseed Meal

2 Tbsps. Red Pepper, Chopped

1 Cup Almond Flour

1/4 Cup Coconut Milk

1 Tsp. Baking Powder

1/2 Tsp. Salt

3 Eggs

1/4 Cup BBQ Sauce

Method

1.   Sift all the dry ingredients (except pork), combine them in one bowl and mix them.

2.   Combine all the wet ingredients (except BBQ sauce) in another bowl, whisk them well and pour in the dry ingredients. Blend them well to make a smooth batter.

3.   Put the batter on to the preheated waffle maker and cook both sides of the waffle until become golden brown.

4.   Mix the pork with 3/4 of the BBQ sauce in a pan and stir fry over medium-low heat for a few minutes.

5.   Transfer the waffles to the serving plate and put a spoonful pork on it. Top with extra BBQ sauce and serve.

15 Cinnamon Roll "Oatmeal"

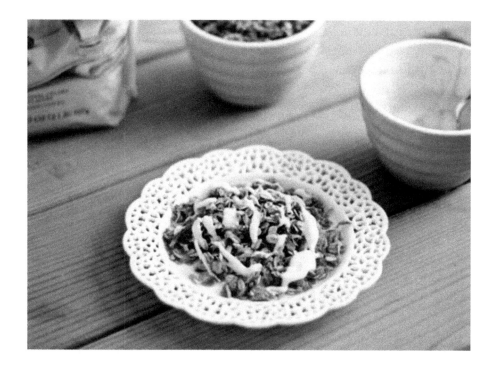

Servings: 6 | **Time**: 35 mins | **Difficulty**: Easy

Nutrients per serving: Calories: 368.83 kcal | Fat: 34.43g | Carbohydrates: 4.08g | Protein: 5.85g | Fiber: 7.44g

Ingredients

1 Cup Pecans, Crushed

1/4 Tsp. Allspice

1/8 Tsp. Xanthan Gum (Optional)

1/4 Tsp. Nutmeg

1/3 Cup Flax Seed Meal

1/2 Tsp. Vanilla

3 Tbsps. Erythritol, Powdered

1/3 Cup Chia Seeds

1 & 1/2 Tsps. Cinnamon

1/2 Cup Cauliflower Rice

3 & 1/2 Cups Coconut Milk

10-15 Drops Liquid Stevia

1/4 Cup Heavy Cream

1/3 Cup Cream Cheese

3 Tbsps. Butter

1 Tsp. Maple Flavor

Method

1.   Chopped the cauliflower rice in a food processor. Toast the crushed pecans on a pan for a minute.

2.   Heat the coconut milk in a saucepan over medium heat and add the cauliflower in it, boil the milk once and let it simmer at low heat. Season with all the spices, add roasted pecans and mix well.

3.   Add the erythritol, stevia and chia seeds, crushed pecans, cream, butter, and cream cheese as well. Mix well and heat until the desired thickness is attained.

4.   Add xanthan gum if you want to make thicker.

16   Maple Pecan Fat Bomb Bars

Servings: 12 | **Time**: 1 hr. 25 mins | **Difficulty**: Easy

Nutrients per serving: Calories: 298.58 kcal | Fat: 29.71g | Carbohydrates: 2.51g | Protein: 4.74g | Fiber: 4.04g

Ingredients

2 Cups Pecan, Toasted & Crushed

1/4 Tsp. Liquid Stevia

1/2 Cup Coconut Oil

1/4 Cup Maple Syrup

1/2 Cup Coconut, Unsweetened & Shredded

1 Cup Almond Flour

1/2 Cup Golden Flaxseed Meal

Method

1.   Preheat the oven at 350 degrees F.

2.   Combine all the ingredients in a bowl and mix well to make a smooth batter.

3.   Put in a casserole dish, press to even it out and bake for 20-25 minutes.

4.   Take out and let cool down to room temperature.

5.   Put in the refrigerator for 1 hour at least, then cut and serve.

17   Ham Cheddar Chive Souffle

Servings: 5 | **Time**: 45 mins | **Difficulty**: Easy

Nutrients per serving: Calories: 406.4 kcal | Fat: 35.85g | Carbohydrates: 3.58g | Protein: 19.63g | Fiber: 0.24g

Ingredients

1 Tbsp. Butter

1/4 Cup Ham Steak, Cooked & Cubed

1 & 1/2 Tsps. Garlic, Minced

1/4 Tsp. Black Pepper

1/2 Tsp. Salt

1/2 Onion, Diced

1 Cup Cheddar Cheese, Shredded

3 Tbsps. Olive Oil

1/2 Cup Heavy Cream

2 Tbsps. Chives, Fresh & Chopped

6 Eggs

Method

1.   Preheat the oven to 400 degrees F.

2.   Heat olive oil in a pan and sauté the onions in it until become soft, then add in the garlic and sauté it too.

3.   Add all the other ingredients except butter in a bowl and mix well until combined.

4.   Brush the butter in ramekins and pour the mixture in them.

5.   Put the ramekins in oven and bake for 20 minutes until golden on top.

18   Maple Sausage Pancake Muffins

Servings: 12 | **Time**: 45 mins | **Difficulty**: Easy

Nutrients per serving: Calories: 160.5 kcal | Fat: 12.88g | Carbohydrates: 2.16g | Protein: 7.6g | Fiber: 2.7g

Ingredients

20 Drops Liquid Stevia

4 Tbsps. Coconut Milk

3/4 Cup Sausage, Ground

1 Tsp. Vanilla Extract

4 Tbsps. Maple Syrup

1 Tsp. Baking Powder

1/4 Tsp. Salt

1/4 Cup Erythritol

2 Tbsps. Psyllium Husk Powder

1 & 1/2 Cups Almond Flour

4 Eggs

Method

1.   Preheat the oven to 350 degrees F.

2.   Crumble the sausage and fry it in a pan until cooked.

3.   Combine all the ingredients, including sausage in a big mixing bowl, first add all the wet ingredients, then wet ingredients with intermittent mixing. Make a smooth batter.

4.   Take a 12-cup muffin tin and divide the mixture among them.

5.   Put in the preheated oven and bake for 20-25 minutes.

6.   Let cool and serve warm.

19 Sausage And Spinach Crustless Quiche

Servings: 10 | **Time**:1 hr. 5 mins | **Difficulty**: Easy

Nutrients per serving: Calories: 429 kcal | Fat: 38g | Carbohydrates: 2g | Protein: 18g

Ingredients

2/3 Cup Baby Spinach, Fresh

1 Cup Heavy Cream

2 Cups Breakfast Sausage Ground

1 Cup Cheddar Cheese, Shredded

1 Cup Cream Cheese, Cubed

6 Eggs

2 Tbsps. Water

Method

1.   Preheat oven to 375 degrees F.

2.　　Cook the ground breakfast sausage in a skillet over medium high heat. Drain out the excess fat and add cream cheese in it.

3.　　Stir well until cream cheese melts completely, then remove from the heat.

4.　　Pour the water in an oven-safe bowl and put the baby spinach in it. Microwave it for 2-3 minutes until spinach wilts and become soft.

5.　　Whisk the eggs and cream together in a bowl. Set aside.

6.　　Take casserole dish, brush it with oil or butter and put the sausage cream cheese mixture at its base.

7.　　Next, spread the spinach on it and sprinkle the shredded cheddar cheese over it.

8.　　At last, pour the egg mixture in it and stir slightly so the egg can reach to the bottom.

9.　　Bake for 35-40 minutes or until the eggs are cooked through.

10.　　Once done, let cool for about 5 minutes, then cut and serve.

20 Bacon, Red Pepper, and Mozzarella Frittata

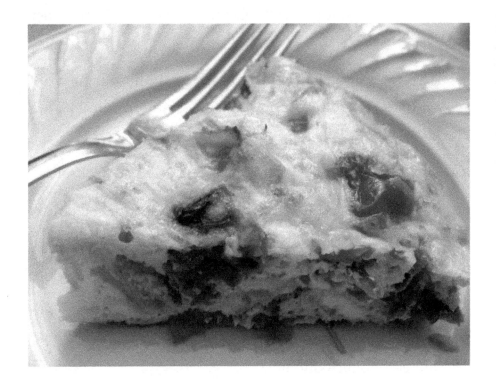

Servings: 6 | **Time:** 25 mins | **Difficulty**: Easy

Nutrients per serving: Calories: 424 kcal | Fat: 34.82g | Carbohydrates: 3.63g | Protein: 22.9g | Fiber: 0.67g

Ingredients

7 Bacon Slices, Chopped

8-9 Eggs

1/4 Cup Parmesan Cheese, Grated

1 Red Bell Pepper, Chopped

Salt, To Taste

1/2 Cup Mozzarella, Fresh & Cubed

1 Tbsp. Olive Oil

1/4 Cup Heavy Cream

Black Pepper, To Taste

1/4 Cup Goat Cheese, Grated

4 Mushroom Caps, Chopped

2 Tbsps. Parsley, Fresh

1/2 Cup Basil, Fresh & Chopped

Method

1.   Preheat the oven to 350F.

2.   Heat the olive oil in a pan and brown the bacon in it. Then add the chopped red pepper and cook it until becomes soft. Add in the chopped mushrooms and sauté it too.

3.   Sprinkle the basil and cubed mozzarella cheese in it, stir well.

4.   Combine the eggs, 1/4 cup parmesan cheese, 1/4 cup heavy cream in a bowl and season with freshly ground black pepper. Whisk them well.

5.   Pour the eggs mixture in the pan as well and stir well to combine everything.

6.   Sprinkle the goat cheese on top and put it in the preheated oven for 6-8 minutes.

7.   Put in the broiler and broil it for 4-6 minutes more.

8.   Let cool for some time and then take the frittata out of the pan. Cut and serve it.

21   Low Carb Cinnamon Orange Scones

Servings: 8 scones with icing | **Time:** 35 mins | **Difficulty:** Easy

Nutrients per serving (scone with extra icing): Calories: 660 kcal | Fat: 60g | Carbohydrates: 7g | Protein: 13g | Fiber: 4.5g

Ingredients

1/4 Cup Butter, Cubed (Unsalted)

2 Eggs

1/4 Tsp. Xanthan Gum

2 Tbsps. Coconut Oil

2 Tbsps. Maple Syrup

1/4 Tsp. Salt

1 Tbsp. Golden Flaxseed

1/4 Cup Erythritol

7 Tbsps. + 1 Tbsp. Coconut Flour

1 & 1/2 Tsps. Baking Powder

2 Tsps. Cinnamon Ground

1/3 Cup Heavy Whipping Cream

1 Tbsp. Orange Zest

1 Tsp. Vanilla Extract

1/4 Tsp. Stevia

20 Drops Liquid Stevia

1 Tbsp. Orange Juice

1/4 Cup Coconut Butter

Method

1.   Preheat the oven to 400 degrees F.

2.   Combine the golden flaxseeds, 7 tbsps. coconut flour, baking powder, cinnamon and orange zest in a bowl and mix well. Add in coconut oil and butter and whisk well.

3.   Whisk the eggs well with sweetener in another bowl until becomes creamy and fluffy. Put the heavy cream, maple syrup, vanilla extract, xanthan gum and remaining coconut flour in it too. Keep mixing until a thick mixture is formed.

4.   Pour this mixture in the flaxseed mixture and mix until a firm dough is formed. Knead the dough into ball and roll it into a circle.

5.   Cut the flattened dough circle into 8 pieces or triangles and put them on a lined baking sheet.

6.   Sprinkle some cinnamon on it if you want and bake for 15-17 minutes in the preheated oven.

7.   Meanwhile combine the icing ingredients in a bowl and mix well.

8.   Once done, take the scones out of the oven and let cool. Top with icing and serve.

22 Maple Pecan Keto Muffins

Servings: 11 | **Time:** 45 mins | **Difficulty**: Easy

Nutrients per serving: Calories: 231.36 kcal | Fat: 21.9g | Carbohydrates: 1.96g | Protein: 5.03g | Fiber: 3.19 g

Ingredients

1 Cup Almond Flour

1/4 Tsp. Liquid Stevia

1/2 Cup Golden Flaxseed

1/2 Tsp. Baking Soda

1 Tsp. Vanilla Extract

1/2 Tsp. Apple Cider Vinegar

3/4 Cup Pecan, Chopped

2 Tsps. Maple Extract

1/2 Cup Coconut Oil

2 Eggs

1/4 Cup Erythritol

Method

1.   Preheat the oven to 325 degrees F.

2.   Combine all the ingredients in a bowl except 1/3 chopped pecans. Mix them well into a smooth batter.

3.   Put the batter in the cups of muffin tin, line with muffin liners.

4.   Sprinkle the reserved pecans on the top and put in the oven.

5.   Bake for 25-30 minutes until completely cooked and let cool before taking out of the muffin tin.

23 Sausage and Cheese Breakfast Pie

Servings: 2 | **Time:** 45 mins | **Difficulty**: Easy

Nutrients per serving: Calories: 900 kcal | Fat: 77.6g | Carbohydrates: 6.86g | Protein: 41.93g | Fiber: 5.45g

Ingredients

2 Tsps. Lemon Juice

5 Egg Yolks

1 & 1/2 Cheddar

Chicken Sausages, Cubed

1/8 Tsp. Kosher Salt

3/4 Cup Cheddar Cheese Grated

1/4 Tsp. Baking Soda

1/4 Cup Coconut Oil

1/4 Tsp. Cayenne Pepper

1/4 Cup Coconut Flour

1/2 Tsp. Rosemary

2 Tbsps. Coconut Milk

Method

1.   Preheat the oven to 350 degrees F.

2.   Sauté the cubed sausages in a pan over medium heat, until cooked through.

3.   Combine all the ingredients in a bowl and mix well to make a smooth and lump free batter.

4.   Brush 2 ramekins with oil or butter and divide the prepared batter in them, filling them about 3/4. Press the sausages into the batter.

5.   Put the ramekins in the oven and bake for 20-25 minutes, or until they become golden brown on top.

24   Pumpkin Cardamom Donut Holes

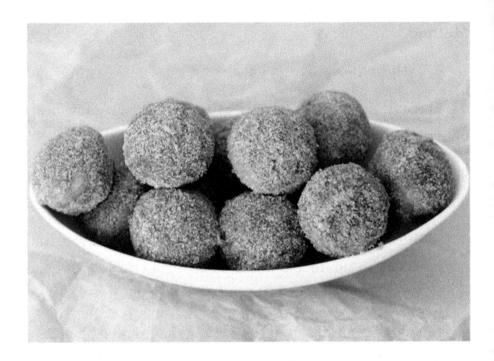

Servings: 18 | **Time**: 45 mins | **Difficulty:** Easy

Nutrients per serving: Calories: 87.68 kcal | Fat: 6.98g | Carbohydrates: 1.78g | Protein: 3.1g | Fiber: 3.15g

Ingredients

2 Tsps. Psyllium Husk Powder

1/2 Cup Pumpkin Puree

1/2 Tsp. Cardamom

1/4 Cup Erythritol/Stevia Blend

1/2 Cup Ricotta Cheese

1/2 Cup Coconut Flour

2 Eggs

1/2 Tsp. Pumpkin Pie Spice

1/4 Cup Butter, Salted

Method

1.   Preheat the oven at 325 degrees F.

2.   Combine all the ingredients in a bowl and mix well to make a smooth and lump free dough.

3.   Knead the dough and make balls with about handful dough, total 18 balls can be made out of it.

4.   Put in the oven and bake for 20-25 minutes or until become light golden brown in color.

5.   Once done, take out and sprinkle some erythritol over them if you want.

25   Pork Rind Caramel Cereal

Servings: 1 | **Time:** 1 hr. 5 mins | **Difficulty:** Easy

Nutrients per serving: Calories: 514 kcal | Fat: 48.38g | Carbohydrates: 2.05g | Protein: 17.12g | Fiber: 1.3g

Ingredients

1/4 Tsp. Cinnamon

2 Tbsps. Butter

2 Tbsps. Heavy Whipping Cream

1 Cup Vanilla Coconut Milk

2 Tbsps. Pork Rinds

1 Tbsp. Erythritol

Method

1.   Take a pan and caramelize the butter in it over medium heat. Once the butter's color changes to brown, take it off the heat and add the erythritol and cream in it.

2.   Mix them well and heat to caramelize the whole mixture.

3.   Once the desired color is attained, take it off the heat and add the pork rinds in it. Break the pork into small pieces to coat them well.

4.   Cover the coated pork rinds in a foil and refrigerate for 20-45 minutes.

5.   Once chilled, if you want to, you can garnish them with nuts serve with milk.

26 Almond Crusted Keto Quiche

Servings: 8 slices | **Time**: 35 mins | **Difficulty:** Easy

Nutrients per serving: Calories: 356.5 kcal | Fat: 30.54g | Carbohydrates: 3.91g | Protein: 16.41g | Fiber: 2.65g

Ingredients

Quiche Crust:

1/4 Cup Olive Oil

1 & 1/2 Cups Almond Flour

1/4 Tsp. Salt

1 Tsp. Oregano, Dried

Quiche Filling:

1/2 Tsp. Pepper

1 Tsp. Mrs. Dash Table Blend

6 Bacon Slices, Diced

1/4 Tsp. Salt

6 Eggs

1 Green Bell Pepper

1 Tsp. Garlic

1 & 1/2 Cups Cheddar Cheese

Method

1.   Preheat the oven to 350 degrees F.

2.   Sauté the bacon pieces in a pan until cooked and put on the paper towels, set aside. Sauté the garlic and green peppers in the same pan. Take out once done.

3.   Combine the eggs, bacon, garlic, green peppers, cheese, Mrs. Dash, salt, and pepper in a container. Mix everything well and set aside.

4.   Combine all the crust ingredients in a bowl and mix well to form a smooth, lump free dough.

5.   Knead the dough and press it in a casserole dish.

6.   Put in the oven and bake for 20 minutes. Take out even when not fully cooked, it can later be cooked with filling. Fill it with the eggs mixture and bake for another 15-18 minutes.

7.   Take out and let cool.

27 Pistachio and Pumpkin Chocolate Muffins

Servings: 8 | **Time**: 55 mins | **Difficulty:** Easy

Nutrients per serving: Calories: 269 kcal | Fat: 23.54g | Carbohydrates: 5.45g | Protein: 7.99g | Fiber: 4.89g

Ingredients

1/4 Tsp. Black Pepper, Ground

4 Eggs

2 Tbsps. Heavy Cream

1/4 Tsp. Kosher Salt

10 Bacon Slices

1/4 Tsp. Mrs. Dash Table Blend

1/2 Cups Cheddar Cheese

2 Tbsps. Bacon Grease

4 Cups Spinach

Method

1.   Preheat the oven to 400 degrees F.

2.   Weave the bacon slices together into a 5x5 bacon weave. Put it on a baking tray.

3.   Bake the bacon weave for 25 minutes in the oven.

4.   In the meantime, whisk the eggs with the cream and set aside.

5.   Once the bacon weave is cooked put it on a paper towel to absorb the grease.

6.   But take the bacon grease from the baking tray and put in a pan. Sauté the spinach in it. Add in the eggs and cream mixture and sprinkle the salt and pepper according to your taste.

7.   Scramble the eggs, and once cooked through, put them on bacon weave. Top with cheese and broil for about 3-4 minutes in the oven.

8.   Let cool for a few minutes and then serve.

29   Almond Flour & Flax Seed Pancakes

Servings: 8 | **Time:** 15 mins | **Difficulty:** Easy

Nutrients per serving: Calories: 225.5 kcal | Fat: 20.42g | Carbohydrates: 2.05g | Protein: 6.43g | Fiber: 5.24g

Ingredients

2 Tbsps. Butter

1/2 Cup Coconut Milk

1/2 Tsp. Nutmeg

2 Tbsps. Erythritol

1/2 Cup Almond Flour

1/2 Cup Flax Seed Meal

1/2 Tsp. Cinnamon

1 Tbsp. Coconut Flour

4 Eggs

5 Tbsps. Coconut Oil

1 Tsp. Baking Powder

1/8 Tsp. Salt

Method

1.   Combine all the ingredients in a bowl (except butter and coconut oil), dry ingredients first, then wet ones. Blend them well to form a smooth batter.

2.   Heat the coconut oil and butter in a pan over medium-high heat. Pour 1/4 Cup batter in it and lower the heat to medium-low.

3.   Cook on both sides for some minutes, until become golden brown and serve with butter and low carb toppings if you want.

30 Low Carb Cinnamon Roll Waffle

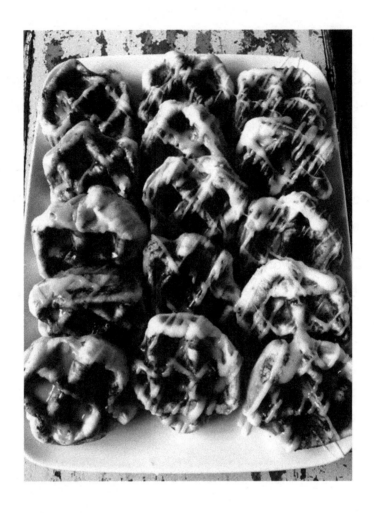

Servings: 1 | **Time:** 25 mins | **Difficulty**: Easy

Nutrients per serving: Calories: 536 kcal | Fat: 44.52g | Carbohydrates: 7.65g | Protein: 24.2g | Fiber: 5.5g

Ingredients

2 Eggs

1/2 Tsp. Vanilla Extract

1/2 Tsp. Cinnamon

6 Tbsps. Almond Flour

1/4 Tsp. Baking Soda

1 Tbsp. Erythritol

Frosting:

2 Tsps. Leftover Batter

1 Tbsp. Heavy Cream

1/4 Tsp. Vanilla Extract

2 Tbsps. Cream Cheese

1/4 Tsp. Cinnamon

1 Tbsp. Erythritol

Method

1.   Combine all the ingredients in a bowl and mix well to make a smooth batter.

2.   Pour the batter in the waffle maker.

3.   In the meantime, whisk together the cream cheese ingredients in a bowl.

4.   Slice the waffle into quarters. Pour the cream cheese filling over the half waffle and spread it evenly.

31   Crispy Stuffed Bacon Baskets

Servings: 4 | **Time**: 1 hr. 15 mins | **Difficulty:** Easy

Nutrients per serving: Calories: 325 kcal | Fat: 26g | Carbohydrates: 1.5g | Protein: 19.8g | Fiber: 0.2g

Ingredients

1 Tbsp. Olive Oil

4 Eggs

2 Tbsps. Heavy Cream

4 Cups Spinach

2/3 Cup Cheddar Cheese

1 Tsp. Pepper

12 Bacon Slices

Method

1.   Preheat the oven to 350 degrees F.

2.   Weave the bacon slices together into a 6x6 bacon weave and cut into quarters.

3.   Put these slices on back of a muffin tray cups at the four corners, that are covered with foil and put it in the oven for 50 minutes.

4.   Once cooked through, take out of the oven and let cool for 10 minutes.

5.   Whisk the eggs and cream in a bowl and set aside.

6.   Sauté the spinach in heated olive oil in a pan and season with black pepper. Once it is cooked, pour in the egg mixture, and cook over low heat.

7.   Put the egg and spinach mixture in the bacon baskets and sprinkle the cheese on top.

8.   Put in the oven and broil until the cheese becomes golden brown. Take out and serve hot.

32 Bacon Wrapped Low Carb Scotch Eggs

Servings: 2 | **Time:** 15 mins | **Difficulty:** Easy

Nutrients per serving: Calories: 477.5 kcal | Fat: 42.36g | Carbohydrates: 2.95g | Protein: 18.91g | Fiber: 3g

Ingredients

1/2 Tbsp. Olive Oil

1 Egg

1 Tbsp. Coconut Oil

2 Tbsps. Coconut Flour

4 Bacon Slices

2 Eggs, Hard Boiled

2 Tbsps. Parmesan Cheese

Method

1.   Combine the coconut flour and parmesan cheese in a bowl and mix them. Set aside.

2.   Whisk 1 egg in another bowl. Set aside.

3.   Wrap each hard-boiled egg in two slices of bacon – one vertical, one horizontal.

4.   Put the bacon-wrapped egg first in the egg mixture and then in the parmesan and coconut flour mixture, again in egg and once again the flour mixture.

5.   Heat the olive oil and coconut oil in a pan over medium-high heat and put the scotch eggs in it. Keep turning it sides to brown from all the sides.

6.   Once browned, lower the heat and fry over it for a while to cook the bacon thoroughly.

7.   When cooked satisfactorily, transfer to paper towel to absorb excess oil.

33 Bacon Crusted Frittata Muffins

Servings: 7 | **Time:** 45 mins | **Difficulty**: Easy

Nutrients per serving: Calories: 467.57 kcal | Fat: 41.83g | Carbohydrates: 2.23g | Protein: 19.35g | Fiber: 0.1g

Ingredients

1/2 Tsp. Cayenne Pepper

18 Bacon Slices

1/2 Tsp. Onion Powder

1/2 Tsp. Celery Salt

7 Eggs

1/2 Tsp. Black Pepper, Ground

1 Cup Cheddar Cheese

4 Tbsps. Heavy Whipping Cream

Method

1.   Preheat the oven to 375 degrees F.

2.   Cut the bacon slices in half and put two to three slices per cup in a muffin tray to cover the cup. Put in the oven and cook for 15 minutes.

3.   Whisk the eggs, cream, and spices in a bowl and set aside.

4.   Put the cheddar cheese in each bacon frittata and pour the egg mixture on top, making sure the egg does not come out.

5.   Bake them for 12-15 minutes more, until their tops begin to brown.

6.   Take out, let cool and serve.

34 Low Carb Mushroom Crustless Quiche

Servings: 6 | **Time:** 40 mins | **Difficulty:** Easy

Nutrients per serving: Calories: 373 kcal | Fat: 34.4g | Carbohydrates: 5g | Protein: 13.32g | Fiber: 0.5g

Ingredients

5 Eggs

1 Cup Mushrooms, Sliced

1 Tbsp. Chives, Snipped

1 & 1/4 Cups Heavy Cream

1/4 Tsp. Black Pepper

3 Tbsps. Butter, Divided

1/2 Cup Gouda Cheese, Smoked & Grated

1/2 Tsp. Salt

1/4 Cup Onion, Minced

1/4 Cup Water

Method

1.   Preheat the oven to 375 degrees F.

2.   Heat 2 tbsps. butter in a pan over medium heat, and sauté mushrooms in it for a few minutes until they become dry. Take out and let cool.

3.   Add the remaining butter in the same pan and once it melts, sauté the onions in it until become soft. Take off the heat.

4.   Beat the eggs with water, cream, salt, and pepper in a bowl until mix well and become frothy.

5.   Spray a pie dish with cooking oil spray and spread 1/3 of the cheese at the base to form a layer. Make a second even layer of the onions, mushrooms, and chives. Spread the egg cream on top and sprinkle the reserved cheese on it.

6.   Put in the oven on a rack placed in the center and bake for 25 minutes or until it is set in the center and golden brown on top.

35 Hunger Buster Low Carb Bacon Frittata

Servings: 8 frittatas | **Time**: 30 mins | **Difficulty**: Easy

Nutrients per serving: Calories: 248.63 kcal | Fat: 19.33g | Carbohydrates: 1.66g | Protein: 16.03g | Fiber: 0.08g

Ingredients

1/2 Cup Half And Half

2 Tsps. Parsley, Dried

1/2 Tsp. Pepper

8 Eggs

1/2 Cup Cheddar Cheese

1/4 Tsp. Salt

1 Tbsp. Butter

1/4 Cup Bacon, Cooked & Chopped

Cooking Spray

Spinach, Sauteed (Optional)

Broccoli, Minced (Optional)

Spring Onion (Optional)

Method

1.   Preheat the oven to 375 degrees F.

2.   Combine all the ingredients in a bowl and mix well.

3.   Spray an 8-cup muffin tin with cooking spray and fill 3/4 of cups with batter.

4.   Put them in the oven and bake for about 15-18 minutes or until become golden.

5.   Take out of the oven and let cool for a while.

36 Low Carb Pumpkin Pancakes

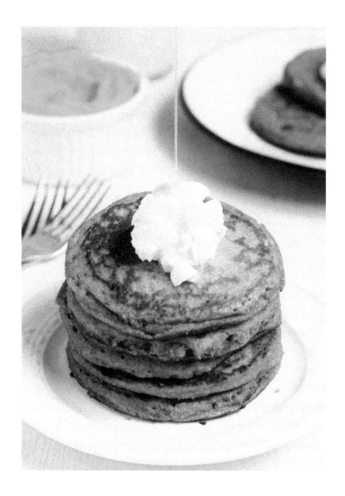

Servings: 8 | **Time:** 35 mins | **Difficulty:** Easy

Nutrients per serving: Calories: 141.18 kcal | Fat: 12.59g | Carbohydrates: 3.53g | Protein: 5g | Fiber: 3g

Ingredients

1 Tsp. Pumpkin Pie Spice

2 Tbsps. Butter

1 Cup Almond Meal

1/4 Cup Sour Cream

1 Tsp. Baking Powder

1/4 Cup Pumpkin Puree

2 Eggs

1/4 Tsp. Salt

Method

1. Combine all the ingredients in a bowl, first dry, then wet and blend until a smooth batter is formed.

2. Grease a skillet with butter and heat it over medium flame.

3. Pour 1/3 cup of the batter in it, for one pancake, and spread with the back of a spoon.

4. Cook both sides of the pancake until they become golden brown. Transfer to a plate once done. Repeat with rest of the batter and serve the pancakes warm.

37   Fluffy Buttermilk Pancakes

Servings: 1 | **Time:** 25 mins | **Difficulty:** Easy

Nutrients per serving: Calories: 422 kcal | Fat: 19.28g | Carbohydrates: 13.01g | Protein: 32.75g | Fiber: 9.8g

Ingredients

1/4 Cup Coconut Flour

1/8 Tsp. Cinnamon

Oil Or Butter, As Needed

2 Eggs, Divided

1 Tsp. Vanilla Extract

1/2 Cup Egg Whites

1 Tbsp. Protein Powder

Salt, To Taste

1 Tsp. Baking Powder

2 Tbsps. Stevia

1/2 Cup Buttermilk

Method

1.   Take the separated egg whites and beat well until become fluffy.

2.   Combine all the other ingredients in a bowl, first dry, then wet and blend until a smooth batter is formed. Add in the egg whites' cream and fold in the batter.

3.   Grease a skillet with butter and heat it over medium flame.

4.   Pour 1/4 cup of the batter in it, for one pancake, and spread with the back of a spoon.

5.   Cook both sides of the pancake until they become golden brown. Transfer to a plate once done.

6.   Repeat this with rest of the batter and serve the pancakes warm.

38   Fast and Easy Coffee Cubes

Servings: 1 | **Time:** 5 mins | **Difficulty:** Easy

Nutrients per serving: Calories: 403 kcal | Fat: 36.86g | Carbohydrates: 6.21g | Protein: 7.7g | Fiber: 5.6g

Ingredients

3 Drops Liquid Stevia

1 Tbsp. Coconut Oil

1 Baking Chocolate Square, Unsweetened

1 Tbsp. Peanut Butter

Method

1.   Put all the ingredient in a ramekin or any other oven safe container and microwave for a minute and stir well until combined and smooth.

2.   Pour the mixture in an ice cubes tray or small cups and freeze.

3.   Whenever you want to use them, just put a cube in your cup and pour the coffee on top. Stir it and serve.

39 Keto Lemon Chia Pudding

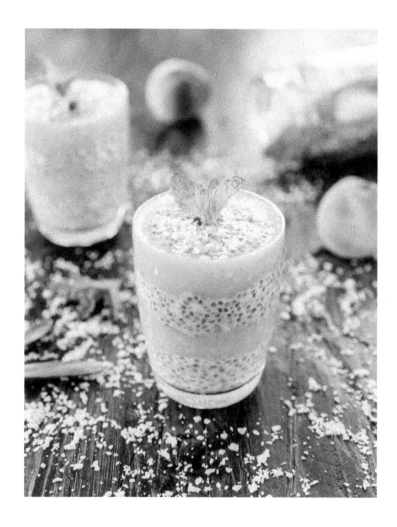

Servings: 4 | **Time:** 5 hrs. | **Difficulty**: Easy

Nutrients per serving: Calories: 343 kcal | Fat: 30.8g | Carbohydrates: 5.9g | Protein: 6.4g | Fiber: 8.75g

Ingredients

2 Tsps. Lemon Zest

1 Cup Coconut Milk

1/2 Cup Heavy Cream

1/2 Cup Chia Seeds

1 Cup Almond Milk, Unsweetened

1/2 Cup Lemon Juice

3 Tbsps. Stevia/Erythritol Blend

Method

1.   Combine all the ingredients in a blender and blend until a smooth mixture is formed.

2.   Put this lemon chia pudding in the serving cups and cover them with cling film.

3.   Put the cups in refrigerator for 5 hours at least and serve later.

40   Two ingredient Pasta

Servings: 1 | **Time:** 5 mins | **Difficulty:** Easy

Nutrients per serving: Calories: 520 kcal | Fat: 34g | Carbohydrates: 11g | Protein: 41g | Fiber: 34g

Ingredients

1 Egg Yolk

1 Cup Mozzarella Cheese, Shredded

Method

1.   Line a baking sheet with parchment paper. Set aside.

2.   Melt the mozzarella cheese in microwave for a minute or two.

3.   Let it cool for a minute and then add the egg yolk in it gradually and mix well.

4.   Once smooth, pour the mixture onto the lined baking sheet, cover it with another piece of parchment paper. Press it with the hand or rolling pin to spread it evenly until a thin dough sheet is formed.

5.   Take off the upper parchment sheet and slice the dough sheet into thin pasta like strips.

6.   Put these pasta strips on a tray and put in the refrigerator overnight.

7.   The next day, boil water in a pan and put the pasta in it for a minute. Drain it and run cold water over it.

8.   Serve with low carb toppings.

41   Low Carb Keto Bagels

Servings: 6 | **Time:** 22 mins | **Difficulty:** Easy

Nutrients per serving: Calories: 245 kcal | Fat: 21g | Carbohydrates: 6g | Protein: 12g | Fiber: 3g

Ingredients

1 & 1/2 Cups Almond Flour

1 Egg

1/4 Cup Cream Cheese

1 & 1/2 Cups Mozzarella Cheese, Shredded

1 Tbsp. Baking Powder

Method

1.   Preheat the oven to 400 degrees F.

2.   Mix the cream cheese and mozzarella cheese in a bowl and microwave it for 30 seconds.

---

3.   Put all the other ingredients in it and whisk well to form a smooth dough. Cover the bowl with cling film and put in the freezer for 10 minutes.

4.   Once the dough is set, knead it and divide it into six pieces. Roll the pieces with hands to form long rods and join their ends to make bagels.

5.   Put the bagels on a lined baking sheet.

6.   Put a rack in the middle of the oven and put the baking sheet on it.

7.   Bake for 12 minutes or until the bagels become golden brown in color.

8.   Take out and let cool and then serve.

42   Steak and Avocado Salad

Servings: 4 | **Time:** 30 mins | **Difficulty:** Easy

Nutrients per serving: Calories: 577 kcal | Fat: 44g | Carbohydrates: 15g | Protein: 32g | Fiber: 8g

Ingredients

2 Cups Cherry Tomatoes, Halved

3 Eggs, Hard-Boiled & Diced

Salt, To Taste

1 Sirloin Steak,

1/2 Inch Thick

2 Tbsps. Oil

2 Hearts Romaine Lettuce, Chopped

Pepper, To Taste

3 Tbsps. Caesar Dressing

2 Avocados, Diced

Method

1.   Take a pan and heat the oil in it over high heat.

2.   Rub the salt and pepper on both sides of the steak and cook it in the pan until it is seared on both sides.

3.   Once done, let cool for 10 minutes, then slice it into strips.

4.   Combine all the ingredients in a bowl, including steak strips and toss well.

5.   Serve and enjoy.

43 Paleo Beef and Veggie Stir-fry

Servings: 6 | **Time**: 35 mins | **Difficulty:** Easy

Nutrients per serving: Calories: 213 kcal | Fat: 11g | Carbohydrates: 4g | Protein: 22g | Fiber: 1g

Ingredients

2 Tbsps. Avocado Oil

1 Tbsp. Ginger, Grated

1 Flank Steak, Sliced

4 Garlic Cloves, Minced

3 & 1/2 Cups Cabbage, Sliced Thinly

2 Tsps. Lime Juice

3 Carrots, Peeled & Sliced

2 Tsps. Coconut Aminos

3 Scallions, Fresh & Minced

Sauce:

1 & 1/2 Tsps. Tapioca Flour

2 Tbsps. Lime Juice

3/4 Cup Coconut Amino

Method

1.   Mix the coconut aminos and lime juice in a bowl and marinate the steak slices with it. Set aside for 10 minutes.

2.   Heat 1 tbsp. avocado oil in a nonstick skillet over medium-high flame and cook the steak slices in it. Once done, take out the steak slices in a bowl.

3.   Add the remaining avocado oil in it and sauté the carrot slices in it until softened, then add the sliced cabbage and stir fry it.

4.   Add in the ginger, garlic, and scallions and fry for half a minute or until fragrant. Mix everything well and add the steak slices as well.

5.   Add in the sauce ingredients as well, mix well and cook for about 1-2 minutes or until a thick sauce is formed. Take off the heat and serve with some chopped scallions on top.

44 Keto Oatmeal

Servings: 1 | **Time:** 5 mins | **Difficulty:** Easy

Nutrients per serving: Calories: 327 kcal | Fat: 27.3g | Carbohydrates: 15.6g | Protein: 11g | Fiber: 11.5g

Ingredients

1/2 Cup Vanilla Almond Milk, Unsweetened

2 Tbsps. Coconut Flakes, Unsweetened

1/2 Tsp. Cinnamon

1 Tbsp. Flax Meal

1/2 Tsp. Vanilla

1/4 Cup Almond Flour

1/8 Tsp. Salt

1/2 Tbsp. Monkfruit

1 Tbsp. Chia Seeds

Method

1.   Combine all the ingredients in a pan except the vanilla and milk, heat them and mix well.

2.   Then pour in the vanilla and milk and boil the mixture over high heat.

3.   After boiling, lower the heat to medium and let it simmer until the mixture thickens to the desired consistency.

4.   Take off the heat and let cool. Add the low carb toppings and enjoy.

45   Low Carb Meatloaf

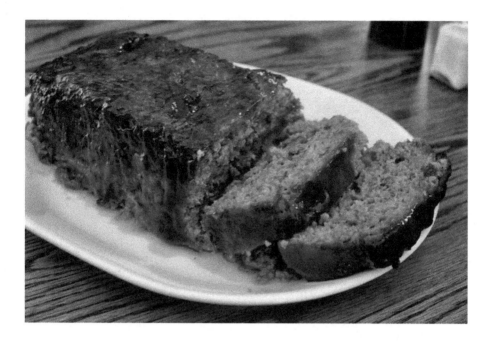

Servings: 6 | **Time:** 1 hr. 10 mins | **Difficulty:** Easy

Nutrients per serving: Calories: 208 kcal | Fat: 12.4g | Carbohydrates: 8.4g | Protein: 17g | Fiber: 1.8g

Ingredients

Sauce:

3 Deglet Noor Dates, Halved

2 Tbsps. Water

1/4 Cup Tomato Paste

1/2 Cup Tomato Sauce

1 Tsp. Onion Powder

1 Tbsp. White Vinegar

1/2 Tsp. Sea Salt

1/2 Tsp. Garlic Powder

For The Meatloaf:

1/4 Cup Green Onion, Sliced

1/2 Tsp. Sea Salt

2 Cups Beef, Ground

1/8 Tsp. Black Pepper

4 Tsps. Coconut Flour

3/4 Cup Green Bell Pepper, Diced

1 Egg

Method

1.   Preheat the oven to 350 degrees.

2.   Make the sauce my heating all its ingredients in a saucepan over high heat. Boil them with constant stirring until combined and thickened to desired consistency.

3.   To further chop the dates, take it off the heat and blend in a food processor or a blender until smooth.

4.   In a bowl combine all the meatloaf ingredients, dry first and wet ones later. Mix them well to make a smooth batter.

5.   Put the batter into a lined loaf pan even it out by pressing it. Pour the sauce over it and spread on top.

6.   Bake for 45-55 minutes or until cooked through.

46   Instant Pot Green Beans

Servings: 4 | **Time:** 16 mins | **Difficulty:** Easy

Nutrients per serving: Calories: 19 kcal | Fat: 0.1g | Carbohydrates: 4.4g | Protein: 1.1g | Fiber: 1.9g

Ingredients

2 Tsps. Garlic, Minced

1 Cup Water

2 Cups Green Beans, Trimmed

1/2 Tsp. Salt

Method

1.   Put all the ingredients into an Instant Pot and stir well. Cover it and seal.

2.   Cook on pressure for 10 minutes.

3.   Drain the beans, sprinkle more salt if needed and serve.

47   Keto Baked Cauliflower Au Gratin

Servings: 6 | **Time**: 45 mins | **Difficulty**: Easy

Nutrients per serving: Calories: 174 kcal | Fat: 12.2g | Carbohydrates: 8.6g | Protein: 9.1g | Fiber: 2.5g

Ingredients

1 Tbsp. + 1 Tsp. Almond Flour

1 & 1/2 Cups Milk

1/4 Tsp. Onion Powder

4 & 1/2 Cups Cauliflower Florets

1/4 Tsp. Garlic Powder

2 Tbsps. Butter

1 Cup Cheddar Cheese, Grated

1 Tbsp. + 1 Tsp. Coconut Flour

1/8 Tsp. Black Pepper

3/4 Tsp. Salt

Method

1.   Put water in a pot and add the salt in it. Boil the water and add cauliflower florets in it. Cook them for about 5-7 minutes or until they become softer. Drain them and soak dry with paper towels.

2.   Heat the butter in a pan over medium-high heat until it melts. Brown the almond and coconut flour in it for about 1 minute and then stir in the milk.

3.   Add in the garlic powder, onion powder, salt, and pepper in it too. Bring it to boil and lower the heat to medium.

4.   Then keep stirring for about 7-8 minutes until the sauce thickens. Take off the heat and add in the 1/2 cup of the grated cheese. Whisk it well to make the sauce smooth.

5.   Preheat the oven to 375 degrees F.

6.   Take an 8×8-inch casserole dish and spread the 1/3 of the sauce at the bottom, Make a layer of cooked cauliflower florets on top, and top it with the remaining sauce.

7.   Sprinkle the remaining cheese on top and put it in the oven.

8.   Bake it for 25-30 minutes or until the cheese becomes golden brown.

48 Low Carb Mock Cauliflower Potato Salad

Servings: 8 | **Time:** 30 mins | **Difficulty:** Easy

Nutrients per serving: Calories: 165 kcal | Fat: 16g | Carbohydrates: 3.8g | Protein: 4.4g | Fiber: 1.7g

Ingredients

4 Eggs, Boiled & Diced

1/4 Cup Red Onion, Diced

Black Pepper, To Taste

Sea Salt, To Taste

5 Cups Cauliflower Florets

1/2 Cup Celery, Sliced Thinly

5 Tsps. Dijon Mustard

2 Tsps. Sea Salt

2 Tsps. Dill Paste

1/2 Tsp. Paprika

1/8 Tsp. Black Pepper

1/2 Cup Mayonnaise

1 Tbsp. Apple Cider Vinegar

Method

1. Put water in a pot and add the salt in it. Boil the water and add cauliflower florets in it. Cook them for about 8 minutes or until they become softer. Drain them and soak dry with paper towels.

2. In the meantime, combine all the dressing ingredients in a bowl and whisk them well.

3. Combine the cauliflower, diced eggs, celery and red onion in a bowl and mix. Add in the dressing and toss the salad well.

4. Cover the bowl and put in the refrigerator for 2 hours at least.

5. Sprinkle the salt and pepper according to your taste and serve.

49   Cauliflower Tabbouleh

Servings: 2 | **Time:** 22 mins | **Difficulty**: Easy

Nutrients per serving: Calories: 660 kcal | Fat: 60g | Carbohydrates: 7g | Protein: 13g | Fiber: 7g

Ingredients

2 Tbsps. Olive Oil

1 Tbsp. Garlic, Fresh & Minced

3 Cups Cauliflower Rice

1 Green Onion

1 Tomato, Diced

2 Tsps. Lemon Juice, Fresh

1/2 Cucumber, Diced

1/2 Tsp. Salt

1/4 Cup Mint Leaves

1/2 Cup Parsley Leaves

Method

1.   Put the cauliflower rice in a bowl and microwave for 3 minutes, covered. Take out, stir once, put back for 3 minutes more. Transfer to a kitchen towel and let cool.

2.   Soak them well with kitchen towel to dry them as much as you can and put in a bowl.

3.   Combine all the other ingredients in the bowl as well and toss well to combine.

4.   Put in the refrigerator for an hour, covered. Serve cold.

50   Keto Banana Bread

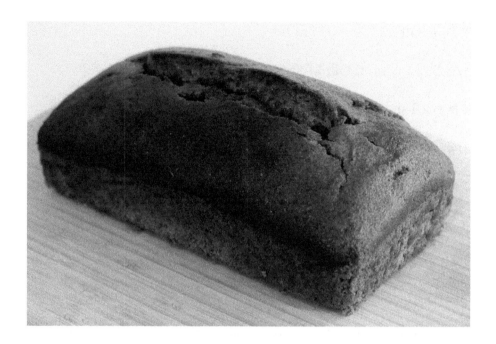

Servings: 2 | **Time:** 1 hr. 10 mins | **Difficulty**: Easy

Nutrients per serving: Calories: 241 kcal | Fat: 22.4g | Carbohydrates: 7.4g | Protein: 7.9g | Fiber: 4.4g

Ingredients

4 Eggs

1/3 Cup Almond Milk, Unsweetened

1 Tsp. Baking Soda

3 Cups Almond Flour

1 Tsp. Salt

1/2 Cup Coconut Oil, Melted

1 & 1/2 Tsps. Cinnamon Powder

1/4 Cup Coconut Flour

1 & 1/2 Tbsps. Banana Extract

2/3 Cup Monkfruit

1 Tbsp. Baking Powder

Method

1.   Preheat the oven to 350 degrees F.

2.   Combine all the ingredients in a bowl, first dry, then wet and blend until a smooth batter is formed.

3.   Line a loaf pan's bottom with parchment paper and brush coconut oil on the sides.

4.   Pour the batter into it and bake for 50 to 60 minutes or until cooked through.

5.   Take out of the oven once done and let cool for an hour. Then, remove gently out of the loaf pan and slice it.

Lightning Source UK Ltd.
Milton Keynes UK
UKHW020653040521
383095UK00001B/62